Qui

Quick Guide to Coagulation Testing

Marisa B. Marques, MD
Associate Professor, Pathology
Division of Laboratory Medicine
School of Medicine
University of Alabama at Birmingham
Birmingham, Alabama

George A. Fritsma, MS, MT(ASCP)
Associate Professor, Pathology and Clinical Laboratory Sciences
University of Alabama at Birmingham
Birmingham, Alabama

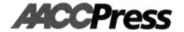

1850 K Street, NW, Suite 625
Washington, DC 20006

4 5 6 7 8 9 0   EB 08

Printed in the United States of America

Library of Congress Cataloging-in-Publication Data

Marques, Marisa B.
   Quick guide to coagulation testing / Marisa B. Marques, George A. Fritsma.
      p. ; cm.
   Includes bibliographical references and index.

   ISBN-13: 978-1-59425-049-1
   ISBN-10: 1-59425-049-9

   1. Blood coagulation tests—Handbooks, manuals, etc.
   [DNLM: 1. Blood Coagulation Tests—methods—Handbooks.   2. Platelet Function Tests—methods—Handbooks. QY 39 M357q 2006]   I. Fritsma, George A.   II. Title.

   RB45.3.M37 2006
   616.1'35075—dc22

                                                              2006007491

Preface

The *Quick Guide to Coagulation Testing* is intended for physicians, nurses, physician assistants, nurse practitioners, medical technologists, and pharmacists, and particularly for residents and students in these professions. The appropriate ordering and interpretation of laboratory assays is an area of medicine often taken for granted. However, the complexity of coagulation testing renders understanding of laboratory results even more critical than in other areas. Lack of awareness of the effect of clinical conditions or the interference of drugs on hemostasis test results may lead to disastrous misinterpretations.

We designed the *Guide* as a speedy reference for anyone who orders, collects, performs, or interprets hemostasis laboratory tests. Its pocket size offers immediate access at the time and location tests are ordered. We included the most common hemorrhagic and thrombotic conditions and emphasize their laboratory evaluation, their treatment with blood products and derivatives (bleeding) or with anticoagulants (thrombosis), and suitable monitoring of treatment by the laboratory. Diseases and their assays are described together so that all conditions may be taken into account when a laboratory workup is warranted.

Although the *Guide* reviews clinical conditions, it should not be used as the sole source to aid in the differential diagnosis of patients; instead, many current references are provided for further reading. Our local experience suggests that the *Guide* is a useful resource for medical professionals. We hope you will find it valuable, too!

Marisa B. Marques
George A. Fritsma

Acknowledgements

The authors wish to express their thanks to...

Lisa Griffin
Karen Waits
Christine Hudson, MT (ASCP)
Cari Reed, MT (ASCP)
Laura Taylor, MT (ASCP)
Patti Tichenor, MT (ASCP)

This booklet is intended as an easily accessible resource to answer commonly asked questions regarding coagulation disorders and testing. It arose from the authors' experiences teaching medical students and physicians at the University of Alabama at Birmingham Hospital through the UAB Coagulation Service. The booklet does not provide a comprehensive review and should be complemented by reading the references, standard textbooks, or published articles. In addition, it does not dictate what constitutes reasonable, appropriate, or best care in specific situations. Thus, the information herein should be used as a general guide to be considered in the context of each patient case. It is not intended for distribution to, or use by, patients.

Some drugs or devices discussed in this book may be either investigational or off-label and not yet approved by the FDA. AACC Press and the University of Alabama at Birmingham Hospital make no warranties concerning the content of this booklet.

Contents

Hemostasis Blood Specimen Management

Hemostasis Blood Specimen Quality

The accuracy of laboratory tests for hemostasis depends on the quality of the blood specimen. Specimens must be properly collected, labeled, stored, and transported. Follow these instructions to maintain specimen integrity and ensure accurate results (1).

Blood Specimen Collection: Whole Blood for Aggregometry, Plasma for Coagulation Testing

1. Establish the identity of the patient.
2. Draw blood into a blue-topped tube that contains 3.2% (0.109 M) sodium citrate anticoagulant. Allow the tube to *fill to the proper level*, determined by the tube's internal pressure reduction, and is usually indicated by the top of the label. Most tubes contain 0.3 mL sodium citrate and draw 2.7 mL of blood. A short draw critically affects the results as there is excess anticoagulant relative to blood volume.
3. Gently invert six times to mix.
4. Label the tube with *patient's full name, medical record number, and the date and time of collection*.
5. *Immediately* transport to the laboratory upright at room temperature. Do not place on ice.

6. Specimens for platelet aggregometry are never centrifuged or refrigerated, and the aggregation test must be performed within three hours.

7. To prepare plasma, centrifuge the stoppered tube at 2500 × g for 10 minutes. *Remember: "g" stands for g-force or relative centrifugal force (RCF), not RPM. Calculate the correct RPM for individual centrifuges using the RCF.*

8. Transfer the plasma with a plastic pipette into a plastic centrifuge tube. Cap the tube and centrifuge it an additional 10 minutes at 2500 × g to obtain *platelet-poor plasma*, which is plasma with a platelet count <10,000 x 10⁹/L. It is *especially important* that plasmas for *lupus anticoagulant and protein S activity testing* be platelet poor.

9. Using care not to disturb the cell button at the bottom, transfer the plasma to another clean plastic tube using a plastic pipette. The tube is sealed and labeled with *patient name, identification number, and date and time of collection.*

10. When plasma testing cannot be completed within four hours of collection, freeze the plasma at −70°C immediately. Specimens should not be frozen in an *ordinary household freezer* nor stored in a *self-defrosting freezer* as the continuous freeze-thaw cycle adversely affects specimen integrity.

11. Ship frozen specimens by overnight delivery with a *minimum of 5 lbs. of dry ice.* Specimens must remain frozen during transport.

12. A properly completed request form with a brief patient history must accompany each specimen. Anticoagulants such as *heparin, warfarin, argatroban, bivalirudin,* and *lepirudin* affect many test results and must be noted on the test request form.

Hematocrit Adjustment for Hemostasis Specimens

The ratio of whole blood to anticoagulant must be 9:1. Standard blue-stopper tubes are calibrated to collect 2.7 mL whole blood to mix with 0.3 mL of 3.2% sodium citrate. When the hematocrit exceeds 55%, the reduced plasma volume necessitates decreasing the volume of sodium citrate using this formula:

$$C \text{ (mL)} = 1.85 \times 10^{-3} \times (100 - \text{HCT [\%]}) \times V \text{ (mL)}$$

where

C = mL of 3.2% sodium citrate to be used

HCT [%] = hematocrit in percent

V = mL of whole blood in tube (2.7 mL)

Thus, to collect 2.7 mL of blood from a patient with a hematocrit of 66.5%:

$$C \text{ (mL)} = 1.85 \times 10^{-3} \times (100 - 66.5) \times 2.7$$

$C \text{ (mL)} = 1.85 \times 10^{-3} \times (33.5) \times 2.7 = 0.17$ mL sodium citrate solution instead of the original 0.3 mL. Therefore, remove 0.13 mL of anticoagulant from the tube before drawing blood.

Therapeutic Ranges and Reference Intervals

Monitoring Heparin and Warfarin	Therapeutic Ranges
Anti-Xa heparin assay: therapeutic low MW heparin, U/mL	0.5–1
Anti-Xa heparin assay: therapeutic Unfractionated heparin, U/mL	0.3–0.7
Anti-Xa heparin assay: prophylactic low MW heparin, U/mL	0.2–0.4
PT warfarin most applications, INR	2–3
PT warfarin, mechanical heart valves, INR	2.5–3.5
PTT unfractionated heparin	Always consult local lab for range
PTT unfractionated prophylactic subcutaneous heparin	Always consult local lab for range

Screening Tests	Reference Intervals
PT, Sec	12.6–14.6
PT, INR	0.93–1.13
PTT, Sec	25–35
TT, Sec	<21

(continued)

Factor Assays	Reference Intervals
Fibrinogen, mg/dL	220–498
Factor II, V, VII, IX, X, XI, XII, %	50–150
Factor VIII, %	50–186
VWF activity (ristocetin cofactor), %	50–166
VWF antigen, %	50–249
HMWK (Fitzgerald), %	65–135
PK (Fletcher), %	65–135

Control Proteins	Reference Intervals
Antithrombin activity, %	78–126
Protein C activity, %	70–140
Protein S activity, %	65–140

Other Assays*	Reference Intervals
Activated protein C resistance, ratio	>1.8
Anti-cardiolipin Antibody IgG, GPL	<12
Anti-cardiolipin Antibody IgM, MPL	<10
D-dimer, ng/mL	110–240
Euglobulin clot lysis time, hours	2–6
Reptilase time, ratio	<1.3

*Reference intervals are laboratory-specific.

Suggested Hemostasis and Coagulation Test Menu

Bleeding Disorders

Intrinsic pathway assay

- Partial thromboplastin time (PTT)

Extrinsic pathway assay

- Prothrombin time (PT) with calculation of the international normalized ratio (INR)

Common pathway assays

- Fibrinogen activity
- Thrombin time (TT)
- Reptilase time (not prolonged by heparin)

Factor assays

- Fibrinogen activity
- Prothrombin (II), V, VII, or X activity (PT-based)
- VIII, IX, XI, or XII activity (PTT-based)
- Qualitative assay for factor XIII deficiency by urea solubility

Coagulation Factor Inhibitors

Follow-up to prolonged PT and/or PTT

- PTT mixing study (incubated)
- PT mixing study (incubated)

Inhibitors

- Lupus anticoagulant
- Factor VIII inhibitor (Bethesda assay)
- Factor IX inhibitor (Bethesda assay)
- Inhibitors to all other factors (rare)

Von Willebrand Disease

Initial profile

- Factor VIII activity
- Von Willebrand factor (VWF) activity—also called ristocetin cofactor
- VWF antigen

Follow-up tests when VWF activity and antigen are discrepant

- Ristocetin response curve
- Von Willebrand factor multimer analysis (electrophoresis)

Platelet Function: Aggregometry

Platelet aggregation and ATP release are measured semiquantitatively using ADP, epinephrine, thrombin, collagen, arachidonic acid, and ristocetin as agonists.

Requires at least 9 mL (three tubes) of whole blood with a minimum platelet count of 100×10^9/L. Specimen must be assayed within 3 hours of collection.

Fibrinolysis Assays

- Fibrinogen activity
- TT
- Reptilase time
- Euglobulin clot lysis time
- Plasminogen activator inhibitor-1 (PAI-1)

Disseminated Intravascular Coagulation (DIC)

- Quantitative D-dimer
- PT
- PTT
- Fibrinogen activity

Anticoagulant Therapy Monitoring

Oral anticoagulants: Warfarin (Coumadin®)

- PT (INR)

Standard unfractionated heparin

- PTT
- Chromogenic anti-Xa heparin assay

Low molecular weight heparin (LMWH, Enoxaparin, Tinzaparin)

- Chromogenic anti-Xa heparin assay

Direct thrombin inhibitors: Argatroban, Lepirudin, Bivalirudin

- PTT

Lupus Anticoagulant (LA) with Follow-Up Assays

Two LA screens are used

- LA sensitive PTT (PTT-LA)
- Dilute Russell viper venom time (DRVVT)

Follow-up assays when either LA screen is positive

- Thrombin time to rule out heparin
- PTT-LA mixing study
- Staclot LA®: PTT confirmatory test using hexagonal phase phospholipid neutralization procedure
- Factor assay if Staclot LA positive
- DRVVT mixing study
- DRVVT confirmatory test

See a full discussion of LA on pages 16–18.

Overview of the Coagulation Mechanism

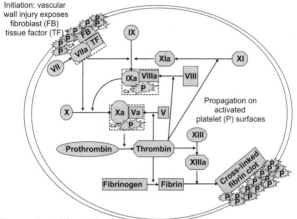

Figure adapted from (2).

- Initiation phase on vascular cells: tissue factor (TF) exposed by injury or inflammation binds activated factor VII (VIIa). TF/VIIa activates factors IX and X (IXa, Xa). The initiation pathway is also known as the extrinsic pathway.
- Propagation phase on activated platelets: thrombin activates factor XI (XIa), which also activates IX. IXa and activated VIII (VIIIa) form VIIIa/IXa, or "tenase complex" that activates X in the presence of calcium on the surface of the platelet plug.
- Xa and activated V (Va) form Va/Xa "prothrombinase complex" that activates prothrombin (II) to form thrombin (IIa), also with calcium and platelets. This is sometimes called the "common" pathway.
- Thrombin cleaves fibrinogen to form a fibrin polymer, and activates factor XIII to cross-link the fibrin strands and stabilize the clot.
- In addition, trace thrombin activates factors XI, VIII, and V for positive feedback of the cascade.

Coagulation Mechanism Controls

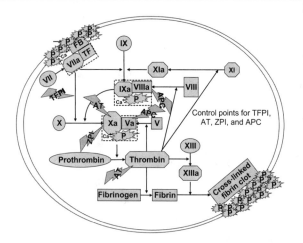

- Tissue factor pathway inhibitor (TFPI) neutralizes TF/VIIa.
- Activated protein C (APC) bound to protein S inactivates Va and VIIIa.
- Protein Z-dependent protease inhibitor (ZPI) inactivates Xa.
- Antithrombin (AT) inactivates multiple steps, especially Xa and thrombin.

Thrombophilia Guidelines

Thrombophilia, or hypercoagulability, implies an increased risk for thrombosis. Thrombophilia may be *congenital* or *acquired*. Thrombosis may be *cardiovascular*, including acute coronary syndromes and peripheral vascular disease; *cerebrovascular*, including transient ischemic attack (TIA) and stroke; or *venous thromboembolic disease*, including deep venous thrombosis (DVT) and pulmonary embolism (PE). Arterial thrombosis is mostly dependent on platelet activation, while venous thrombosis may be caused by coagulation system abnormalities in addition to stasis and/or vascular injury (Virchow's triad). This discussion focuses on risk factors for venous thromboembolism (3).

Why Perform Thrombophilia Testing?

- To establish the pathologic basis of a thrombotic event and provide the opportunity to communicate etiologic factors to patients.
- To influence the duration of therapy following a thrombotic episode.
- To offer prophylaxis for high-risk patients during periods of potentially increased stimulus—see "Circumstantial Thrombophilia Risk Factors" below.
- To alert the patient's kindred to the presence of inherited risk factors.
- To determine the need for alternative laboratory testing when a condition affects the primary testing mode such as heparin

monitoring in patients with a prolonged PTT due to lupus anticoagulant.

Refer to the acute thrombophilia test profile on page 16 for recommended assays to order during thrombotic episodes.

Circumstantial Thrombophilia Risk Factors

- Age, previous thrombosis, smoking
- Pregnancy, oral contraceptives, hormone replacement therapy
- Immobilization: travel, bedfast, wheelchair, sedentary lifestyle
- Diet, obesity affecting lipids and immobilization
- Orthopedic surgery, neurosurgery, trauma, fractures
- Blood group non-O with increased VWF and factor VIII

Disease-Related Thrombophilia Risk Factors

- Autoimmune disorders: systemic lupus erythematosus, antiphospholipid syndrome
- Malignancies: adenocarcinoma, chronic myelogenous leukemia, essential thrombocythemia, polycythemia vera, acute promyelocytic leukemia, acute monoblastic leukemia
- Congestive heart failure and other cardiovascular diseases
- Paroxysmal nocturnal hemoglobinuria
- Chronic inflammatory diseases leading to elevated factor VIII and fibrinogen

Circumstances That Suggest a Thrombophilia Workup

- Thrombosis before 40–50 years of age
- Unprovoked thrombosis at any age
- Recurrent thromboses at any age

- Thrombosis in an unusual site such as cerebral, mesenteric, portal, or hepatic veins
- Positive family history for thrombosis
- Thrombosis during pregnancy, oral contraceptives, or hormone replacement therapy
- Unexplained abnormal laboratory test such as prolonged PTT

Complete Thrombophilia Laboratory Test Profile

The following series of assays may be ordered if the patient is not taking or has not taken an anticoagulant such as warfarin or heparin for at least 10 days, and does not have current thrombosis.

- Activated protein C resistance (APCR)
  - Follow up with factor V Leiden mutation molecular assay when the APCR ratio is below the cutoff, indicating resistance
- Lupus anticoagulant testing
- Anticardiolipin antibodies (ACA, ACL): IgG and IgM
- Antithrombin activity
  - Follow up with antithrombin antigen assay if activity is consistently below the reference limit
- Fasting homocysteine
- Factor VIII activity
- Protein C activity
  - Follow up with protein C antigen assay if activity is consistently below the reference limit
- Protein S activity
  - Follow up with free and total protein S antigen if activity is consistently below the reference limit
- Prothrombin 20210 mutation molecular assay

Selective Thrombophilia Test Profile

The following assays are the only ones that can be interpreted when the patient is currently experiencing a thrombotic event, is currently taking anticoagulants, or has had either in the last 10–14 days.

- Activated protein C resistance (APCR)
  - Follow up with factor V Leiden mutation molecular assay when the APCR ratio is below the cutoff, indicating resistance
- Fasting homocysteine
- Anticardiolipin antibodies (ACA, ACL): IgG and IgM
- Prothrombin G20210A mutation molecular assay

Lupus Anticoagulant Testing Algorithms

Lupus Anticoagulant Flow Chart
Prolonged Dilute Russell Viper Venom Time (DRVVT)

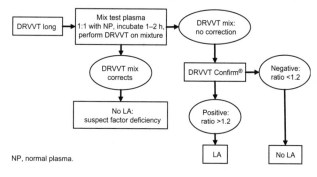

NP, normal plasma.

Lupus Anticoagulant Flow Chart
Prolonged Lupus Anticoagulant-Sensitive PTT (PTT-LA) and Staclot LA

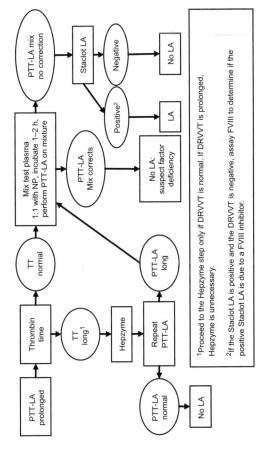

[1]Proceed to the Hepzyme step only if DRVVT is prolonged. If DRVVT is normal, Hepzyme is unnecessary.

[2]If the Staclot LA is positive and the DRVVT is negative, assay FVIII to determine if the positive Staclot LA is due to a FVIII inhibitor.

17

Lupus Anticoagulant (LA) Testing

Because LA is an IgG immunoglobulin that binds protein-binding phospholipids, it is identified by its ability to prolong clot-based assays designed with a limited supply of reagent phospholipid. Testing requires a series of steps starting with at least two assays that are known to be affected by LA (4). Laboratories may choose to employ a low phospho-lipid PTT reagent designed to detect LA (PTT-LA) and the dilute Russell viper venom time (DRVVT) test. Since unfractionated heparin affects the PTT-LA, a prolonged result should be followed by a thrombin time to detect heparin. If the latter is prolonged, the sample is treated with Hepzyme® and the PTT-LA repeated. The DRVVT reagent has a heparin neutralizer but is affected by warfarin.

- When heparin is ruled out, PTT-LA should be repeated in a 1:1 mixture of patient and normal plasma incubated for at least 1 hour at 37°C (mixing study). The same applies to a prolonged DRVVT. If the result of one or both mixing studies is prolonged to more than 10% above the normal plasma alone (lack of correction), LA is likely.
- LA is confirmed by correction of the prolonged PTT-LA and/or DRVVT with a high phospholipid reagent such as Staclot LA and DRVVT-confirm and ratio. If LA affects only the PTT-LA, rule out a factor VIII inhibitor by performing a factor VIII activity level.

  See page 10 for a recommended summary of LA tests.

Anti-Cardiolipin Testing (ACL)

ACLs of IgG or IgM isotype are measured in immunologic assays (ELISA) and do not prolong clot-based tests. A medium or high titer result on two or more consecutive occasions at least 12 weeks apart is evidence for chronicity and possible antiphospholipid syndrome.

Antiphospholipid Syndrome (APS)

Antiphospholipid antibodies (APLs) in the form of LA or ACLs are found in 5% of unselected individuals, and 2% remain on repeat testing (5). They are also found in 10–50% of people with autoimmune disorders. APS is the most common acquired thrombophilic condition with a relative risk of thrombosis for people with primary APLs of 1.6 to 3.2. APS is diagnosed when a patient has a history of thrombosis or pregnancy complications *and* a positive LA or anticardiolipin antibody that persists for 12 weeks.

Vascular thrombosis

One or more clinical episodes of arterial or venous thrombosis in any tissue confirmed by imaging, Doppler, or histopathology without evidence of vessel wall inflammation may be evidence for APS.

Obstetric morbidity

APS is suspected if a patient has a history of fetal death at or after 10 weeks' gestation, premature birth at or before 34 weeks' gestation, or three or more consecutive spontaneous abortions before the 10th week of gestation (6).

Risk of Venous Thromboembolism in Acquired Thrombophilia (7)

• Femoral and tibial fractures	80%
• Hip, knee, GYN, prostate surgery	50%
• Adenocarcinoma	20×
• Chronically elevated factor VIII	6×
• Oral contraceptives (30 µg)	4–6×
• Pregnancy	3–5×
• Hormone replacement (5 µg)	2–4×
• Homocysteinemia due to vitamin deficiency	2–7×
• Chronic APL without a known autoimmune disorder	1.6–3.2×

Prevalence of Congenital Thrombophilia

Factor	General Population	People with Thrombosis
• APCR: factor V Leiden mutation (8,9)	3–8% of Caucasians	20–25%
• Prothrombin G20210A (8,9)	2–3% of Caucasians	4–8%
• Antithrombin deficiency (8,9)	1 in 2000–5000	1–1.8%
• Protein C deficiency (8,9)	1 in 300	2.5–5.0%
• Protein S deficiency (8,9)	Unknown	2.8–5.0%
• Hyperhomocysteinemia (8,9)	11%	13.1–26.7%

Risk of Venous Thromboembolism in Congenital Thrombophilia

Factor	Odds of Thrombosis
• APCR: heterozygous factor V Leiden mutation (8,9)	3×
• APCR: homozygous factor V Leiden mutation	18×
• Prothrombin G20210A heterozygotes (8,9)	2–4.8×
• Antithrombin deficiency heterozygotes (8,9)	10–20×
• Protein C deficiency heterozygotes (8,9)	6.5×
• Protein S deficiency heterozygotes (8,9)	1.6–11.5×

Anticoagulant Therapy Monitoring Guidelines

Warfarin (Coumadin®) (10,11)

Indications for warfarin

- Treatment of arterial and venous thrombosis to prevent clot propagation
- Prevention of thromboembolic disease in thrombophilia, atrial fibrillation, mechanical heart valves, and high-risk surgery

Mechanism of action of warfarin

- Prevents γ-carboxylation of the vitamin K-dependent factors II, VII, IX, and X, and proteins C, S, and Z, slowing thrombin production

Dosage of warfarin

- 5–10 mg/day with no loading dose. Warfarin must be monitored due to unpredictable pharmacokinetics.
- Affected by many drugs and dietary variation
- Requires 4–7 days to reach therapeutic levels. To achieve immediate anticoagulation, overlap with heparin for several days until INR is therapeutic for at least two consecutive days.

Laboratory monitoring: The INR

PT generates the INR by this formula:

$$INR = (Patient\ PT/MRI\ PT)^{ISI}$$

where

- INR = international normalized ratio
- MRI = geometric mean of reference interval (specific for each laboratory)
- PT = prothrombin time in seconds
- ISI = international sensitivity index supplied by reagent manufacturer

Target INRs (10)

- Therapy or prophylaxis for venous thrombosis: 2.0–3.0 (including patients with APS)
- Post-recurrence of thrombosis during therapeutic INR: 2.5–3.5
- Mechanical heart valves: 2.5–3.5
- Post-myocardial infarction with high risk of recurrence: 1.5 (11)

Laboratory monitoring sequence

- Daily PT until INR is therapeutic at least 24 hours apart
- Check PT twice a week for 2 weeks, then once a month until therapy is complete

Managing Warfarin Overdose (10)

INR	Bleeding	Intervention
Above therapeutic range but less than 5	No significant bleeding	Lower or omit dose, monitor INR more frequently
Between 5 and 9	No significant bleeding	Omit warfarin doses, monitor INR more frequently, consider oral vitamin K ($\leq$ 5mg) if high risk for bleeding (surgery)
Greater than 9	No significant bleeding	Stop warfarin, give oral vitamin K (5–10 mg), monitor INR more frequently
Any INR	Serious bleeding	Stop warfarin, give vitamin K SQ (10 mg), may repeat every 12 hours, give fresh frozen plasma (FFP) or prothrombin complex concentrate (may use recombinant factor VIIa)
	Life-threatening bleeding	Same as serious bleeding, except stronger indication for recombinant factor VIIa

Standard Unfractionated Heparin (UFH) (12)

Indications for UFH

- Treatment or prevention of arterial and venous thrombosis

Mechanism of action

- Increases the inhibitory effect of antithrombin on the serine proteases thrombin, IXa, Xa, XIa, and XIIa with greatest effect upon thrombin
- UFH clearance varies by individual and requires routine monitoring

Usual dosage for therapy of thrombosis

- 80 IU/kg bolus, 8 IU/kg/h IV started concurrently with warfarin
- Discontinue after 5 days if the INR has been therapeutic for at least 24 hours

Laboratory monitoring: PTT

- Assay 4–6 hours after bolus dosage and every 24 hours thereafter; if dose adjustment is needed, 6 hours after changing IV infusion
- PTT therapeutic range must be determined in each laboratory based upon the heparin anti-Xa assay range of 0.3–0.7 U/mL
- Target PTT interval varies with reagent lot and instrument used for testing

Laboratory monitoring: platelet count

- Daily platelet count should be checked to detect heparin-induced thrombocytopenia (HIT)
- If count drops 30–50%, consider HIT, withdraw heparin, start alternative anticoagulant, order confirmatory test for HIT (see below) (13)

Overdose of UFH

- Stop heparin and monitor PTT. Heparin half-life is approximately 30 minutes. If bleeding is severe, consider protamine sulfate (1 mg/ 100 units heparin)
- FFP does not reverse heparin effect

Heparin-Induced Thrombocytopenia with Thrombosis (HIT) (13)

Up to 10% of patients receiving unfractionated heparin develop an IgG immunoglobulin directed at heparin-bound platelet factor 4 (PF4). In a variable percentage of these patients, the immune complex of IgG-PF4-heparin activates platelets through their Fc receptor and causes a drop in platelet count due to platelet aggregation. Consequently, the patient may develop arterial and/or venous thrombosis, a major source of morbidity and mortality. A decrease in platelet count of 30–50% during heparin therapy (more commonly IV but could also be caused by SQ low molecular weight heparin), even when the count remains within the normal range, may signal the onset of HIT. Laboratory confirmation consists of an immunoassay for the anti-heparin-PF4 antibody. This assay may require several hours and yields a relatively high false positive rate, thus it is confirmatory but not diagnostic. When clinical suspicion is high, heparin should be replaced with a direct thrombin inhibitor such as lepirudin or argatroban until the clinical situation is elucidated. On the other hand, even a negative test result for PF4 antibodies may still be consistent with HIT and a repeat test may be indicated in the right clinical setting (unexplained thrombocytopenia with or without thrombosis).

Low Molecular Weight Heparin (LMWH): Enoxaparin, Tinzaparin, Dalteparin

Indications for LMWH

- Prevention or treatment of thromboembolic disease

Mechanism of action

- Increases the inhibitory effect of antithrombin on Xa and thrombin with greatest effect on Xa
- LMWH renal clearance is predictable and monitoring is not often necessary

Dosage for Enoxaparin

- Prophylaxis: 40 mg SQ once a day (for morbidly obese, may need 60 mg)
- Therapeutic: 1 mg/kg q12h (maximum of 150 mg)
- For special situations, see reference 12.

Fondaparinux (Arixtra®, Pentasaccharide)

Dosage

- Prophylaxis: 2.5 mg SQ once a day
- Therapeutic: Not established

Laboratory Monitoring of LMWH and Fondaparinux

- Use chromogenic anti-Xa heparin assay
- PTT reagents vary in their sensitivity to LMWH or pentasaccharide
- Assay not necessary in uncomplicated treatment situations
- Assay needed for infants, children, obese or underweight patients, those with renal disease, those on long-term treatment, pregnant patients, or those having unexpected bleeding or thrombosis

- Target for prophylaxis: 0.2–0.4 anti-Xa U/mL (four hours post-injection)
- Target for therapy: 0.5–1.0 anti-Xa U/mL
- Pentasaccharide target: 0.14–0.19 mg/L (not widely available in clinical laboratories)

Direct Thrombin Inhibitors (DTIs): Argatroban and Lepirudin (13)

DTI indications

- Substitute a DTI for heparin when HIT is suspected or confirmed. Even when HIT's only manifestation is thrombocytopenia and heparin is stopped, risk of thrombosis in subsequent 30 days approaches 50%, unless alternative anticoagulant is used.

DTI dosages

- Lepirudin: 0.4 mg/kg slowly IV, then 0.15 mg/kg continuous infusion for 2–10 days depending on indication
- Argatroban: 2 µg/kg/min IV

DTI half-lives

- Lepirudin: 20 minutes (cleared by the kidneys)
- Argatroban: 39–51 minutes (cleared in the liver)

Laboratory monitoring of DTIs

- PTT is used to prevent bleeding or thrombosis. Neither drug has a known antidote.
- Lepirudin: collect blood 4 hours after initial dosage, adjust dosage to PTT 1.5–3.0 × mean of reference interval
- Argatroban: collect blood 2 hours after initial dosage, adjust dosage to PTT 1.5–3.0 × mean of reference interval
- Do not start in patients with prolonged baseline PTT

- In HIT, warfarin may be introduced when platelet count starts to increase but DTIs should be continued until platelet count normalizes. After 4–5 days of warfarin, if platelet count is normal and PT is therapeutic, stop DTI for a few hours and recheck INR. If the INR is between 2 and 3, it is safe to discontinue DTI.

Guidelines for the Management of Bleeding

Hemorrhage and Coagulopathy (14)

Most bleeding stems from local tissue injuries, not coagulopathies. Suspect a coagulopathy when bleeds issue from multiple sites or are spontaneous, inappropriately excessive, or recurrent. Most coagulopathies are acquired and may be traced to a drug or an underlying systemic disorder.

Systemic (mucocutaneous) bleeding

Petechiae, easy bruising, epistaxis, hematemesis, or menorrhagia characterize systemic mucocutaneous bleeds. Systemic bleeds usually imply a defect in primary hemostasis: thrombocytopenia, a platelet qualitative abnormality, von Willebrand disease, or a vascular disease such as scurvy.

Anatomic (soft tissue) bleeding

Anatomic bleeds affect joints, muscles, the peritoneum, or the central nervous system. Anatomic bleeds usually imply the impairment of secondary hemostasis, meaning coagulation factor deficiencies. Patients often have multiple coagulation factor defects or are taking medications that interfere with hemostasis.

Acquired vs. congenital bleeding

Acquired bleeds are seen most often in adults, follow identifiable events or an underlying disorder, and show no familial pattern. Congenital bleeds, with the classic example of hemophilia, usually occur in children and may be spontaneous, recurrent, or accompanied by positive family history. When a coagulation disorder is suspected, treatment may include FFP, cryoprecipitate, platelet transfusion, or specific coagulation factor concentrates. However, treatment should only be started after the cause is known. In emergencies, at least collect blood for laboratory assays prior to transfusing any products.

Tests Used to Establish Presence of Coagulopathies

Perform these tests when bleeding suggests a coagulopathy in the absence of anticoagulant therapy.

Prothrombin time (PT)

If the PT is prolonged, especially more than $1.5 \times$ the mean of the reference interval, suspect single or multiple deficiencies of the "extrinsic" and "common" factors prothrombin, fibrinogen, V, VII, or X. The factor with the greatest impact on the PT is VII (responsible for the "initiation" of activation).

Partial thromboplastin time (PTT)

If the PTT is prolonged, especially more than $1.5 \times$ the mean of the reference interval, suspect single or multiple deficiencies of the "intrinsic" and "common" factors prothrombin, fibrinogen, V, VIII, IX, X, or XI. Deficiencies of the "contact" factors XII, Fletcher (prekallikrein), or Fitzgerald (high molecular weight kininogen, HMWK) also prolong the PTT but are not associated with bleeding. PTT results > 200 seconds indicate heparin contamination until proven otherwise.

Interpreting PT and PTT Results

PT and PTT results in combination are useful when the patient is not on an anticoagulant and when bleeding suggests a coagulopathy. Rule out unreported heparin in the laboratory using the thrombin time, which is prolonged to >21 seconds when heparin is present.

PT	PTT	Acquired Disorder	Congenital Disorder
Long	Normal	Liver disease or vitamin K deficiency[a]	Factor VII deficiency[b]
Normal	Long	Acquired factor VIII inhibitor[c]	Factor VIII, IX, or XI deficiency[d]
Long	Long	DIC, liver disease, acquired factor deficiency (amyloidosis), LA[e]	Fibrinogen[f], prothrombin, factor V, or factor X deficiency
Normal	Normal	Thrombocytopenia, qualitative platelet disorder, acquired von Willebrand disease	Mild factor deficiency(ies), mild von Willebrand disease, factor XIII deficiency[g]

[a]To distinguish liver disease from vitamin K deficiency, assay factors V and VII. If only VII is deficient, suspect vitamin K deficiency; if both are deficient, suspect liver disease.

[b]Congenital factor VII deficiency is rare and causes childhood bleeding. The intensity of bleeding correlates poorly with VII activity.

[c]Acquired factor VIII inhibitor is a rare autoimmune disease called "acquired hemophilia" with severe bleeding (15). The inhibitor is identified using the PTT mixing study and the factor VIII assay and is measured in Bethesda units.

[d]Factors VIII and IX deficiencies are X-linked and are almost always diagnosed in childhood (unless mild). They are called hemophilia A and hemophilia B, respectively. Factor XI deficiency (hemophilia C) is autosomal recessive and is most common in Ashkenazi Jews. However, it can occur in any ethnic group. Factor XI activity correlates poorly with bleeding intensity.

[e]LA is seldom associated with bleeding unless it binds to and neutralizes prothrombin.

[f]Fibrinogen deficiency prolongs both PT and PTT, but only when the concentration is <100 mg/dL. Deficiencies of factors V, X and prothrombin are rare.

[g]Factor XIII deficiency is established using the *urea solubility test*.

PTT Mixing Study

When the PTT is prolonged beyond the upper limit of the reference interval, the patient's plasma should be mixed 1:1 with reagent normal plasma and the PTT repeated.

- If the PTT corrects to within 10% of the reagent normal plasma PTT and the patient is bleeding, suspect a coagulation factor deficiency. Proceed with factor levels, assaying the most likely one first.
- If the PTT fails to correct, and the patient is not bleeding, suspect LA. Proceed with LA confirmation as detailed under "Thrombophilia Guidelines."
- Some LAs and specific factor inhibitors (such as factor VIII) are time- and temperature-dependent. If the PTT corrects to within 10% of the normal plasma PTT, repeat the mixing study by incubating the mixture for 1 to 2 hours at 37°C. If the incubated PTT fails to correct, there is an inhibitor in the sample.

Heparin interferes with mixing studies and prevents correction. Rule out unreported heparin using the thrombin time, which is prolonged >21 seconds when heparin is present.

Blood Components

Treating multiple factor deficiencies with fresh frozen plasma (FFP)

FFP is the plasma from a unit of whole blood separated by centrifugation and frozen within 8 hours of collection. It is stored at −18°C or colder for up to 12 months, thawed at 30–37°C and kept at 1–6°C for no longer than 24 hours after thawing begins. FFP contains an average of 1 U/mL of each coagulation factor, including the labile factors V and VIII. FFP is primarily used to treat the bleeding of acquired multiple factor deficiencies that occurs in liver disease, vitamin K deficiency, DIC, and massive transfusion. Less frequently, it may be used to treat the rare congenital single factor deficiencies of prothrombin, V, VII, X, or XI, or deficiencies of proteins C or S. FFP may be used for immediate short-term reversal of over-anticoagulation with warfarin. *However, because of its 3- to 5-hour half-life, factor VII is difficult to replace using FFP without causing volume overload.* Thus, vitamin K and FFP are indicated in patients who have a high INR and are bleeding. FFP is the replacement fluid of choice in therapeutic plasma exchange for thrombotic thrombocytopenic purpura (TTP) and hemolytic uremic syndrome (HUS).

A dose of 10–20 mL of FFP/kg of body weight will increase any factor level by 20–30%. Frequency of transfusion depends on the half-life of the deficient factor(s). FFP is not indicated unless the PT or PTT is >1.5 × the mean of the normal range, there is evidence of factor deficiencies, and the patient is bleeding. FFP should not be used as a volume expander, or to "correct" a mildly prolonged PT or PTT. A patient may have a mildly prolonged PT or PTT and yet have hemostatically stable levels of coagulation factors.

Treating fibrinogen and factor XIII deficiency with cryoprecipitate (CRYO)

CRYO is the protein precipitate left after FFP is thawed at 4°C and the supernatant liquid plasma is removed. CRYO is refrozen and stored at −18°C or lower for up to 12 months. After thawing at 30–37°C, it is kept at 20–24°C for no longer than 6 hours, or if pooled, no longer than 4 hours. A unit contains at least 80 U of factor VIII, 150–250 mg of fibrinogen, 50–75 U of factor XIII, and VWF.

CRYO is the only source of concentrated fibrinogen available, and is most commonly transfused to replace acquired fibrinogen deficiencies due either to DIC or thrombolytic therapy, or for congenital hypofibrinogenemia or dysfibrinogenemia. A fibrinogen concentration of 50–100 mg/dL is considered hemostatically effective, and can be achieved by infusing one unit of CRYO/7 kg of body weight. Fibrinogen has a half-life of 100–150 hours.

CRYO is also used to treat the rare congenital or acquired deficiency of factor XIII. Factor XIII has a long half-life, 7–12 days, so the recommended treatment for factor XIII deficiency is one unit of CRYO/10 kg every 7 days.

Disseminated Intravascular Coagulation (DIC) Profile (16)

DIC is generalized activation of coagulation secondary to systemic conditions such as septicemia, carcinoma, severe inflammation, or pregnancy complications. The presence of a high concentration of D-dimer, often >20,000 ng/mL, is the *sine qua non* criterion for DIC, as the elevation reflects increased fibrin production and breakdown. In acute DIC, activation of the tissue factor (extrinsic or initiation) pathway decreases factors II, VII, IX, and X, prolonging the PT and PTT. However, an increase in factor VIII production coupled with VWF released from the endothelium may make the PTT less useful than the PT in laboratory diagnosis of DIC. The PT is also expected to be prolonged before the PTT because it depends on the factor VII level, which has a half-life of 3–5 hours.

DIC treatment issues

The most important aspect of treating DIC is to remove the underlying cause of the syndrome. Secondly, it is crucial to maintain the blood pressure and to correct electrolyte imbalances to improve tissue oxygenation. Transfuse FFP, CRYO, and platelets if there are signs of ineffective hemostasis, such as profuse oozing or frank bleeding. Results of PT, PTT, fibrinogen, and platelet count should guide therapy. High D-dimer levels and increased fibrinolysis suppress platelet function and add to defective hemostasis.

Assays Useful in the Diagnosis of DIC

Assay	Expected Results in DIC
Quantitative D-dimer	Significantly above the upper limit of reference interval
	○ Single most important assay to establish DIC
	○ In compensated DIC, D-dimer may be the only abnormal test
PT	Usually prolonged (even before PTT becomes prolonged)
PTT	Usually prolonged above upper limit of reference interval
Fibrinogen	Low; but may be normal or high due to acute phase reaction; sequential measurements are helpful
Complete blood count with platelet count	Anemia with schistocytes, thrombocytopenia*

*Low platelet count reflects significant consumption but count may be near normal due to marrow response

Von Willebrand Disease (VWD) (17)

VWD is a deficiency or abnormality of plasma VWF, a 5–20 million Dalton multimeric protein essential to platelet adhesion. VWF is also the plasma carrier of coagulation factor VIII. VWD affects 1–2 % of the general population. Clinicians must differentiate the various types and subtypes of VWD before establishing treatment using a series of laboratory assays.

VWD Clinical Manifestations and Pathology

VWD Type	Bleeding	Pathology	Inheritance Pattern and Incidence
1	Mild to moderate	Various mutations throughout VWF gene	Autosomal dominant; 75–80%
2A	Moderate to severe	Mutation in VWF-protease cleavage site	Autosomal dominant or recessive; 10–15%
2B	Moderate to severe	Gain of function mutation in GPIb binding site	Autosomal dominant; 5%
2M	Moderate	Loss of function mutation in GPIb binding site	Autosomal dominant or recessive; infrequent
2N	Moderate	Mutation in factor VIII binding site	Autosomal recessive; infrequent
3	Severe	Decreased mRNA expression	Autosomal recessive; rare

Acquired VWD

Acquired VWD is multifactorial and may arise because of an antibody to VWF, reduced VWF production, or increased turnover. It is associated with monoclonal gammopathy of unknown significance (MGUS), non-Hodgkin's lymphoma, multiple myeloma, solid tumors, hypothyroidism, and sodium valproate and ciprofloxacin among other causes/drugs.

VWD Laboratory Profile*

VWD Type	Primary Assays			Follow-Up Assays	
	VWF Antigen	Ristocetin Cofactor (VWF Activity)	Factor VIII Activity	Ristocetin-Induced Platelet Aggregation	VWF Multimers by Gel Electrophoresis
Normal	50–150%*	50–166%*	50–186%	Positive using 1 mg ristocetin	Normal distribution
1	Mildly decreased	Mildly decreased	Mildly decreased	Variable	Normal distribution
2A	Mildly decreased or normal	Lower than antigen	Normal	Variable	Absence of high and intermediate molecular weight multimers
2B	Mildly decreased or normal	Lower than antigen	Normal	Positive using 1 and 0.5 mg ristocetin	Absence of high molecular weight multimers
2M	Mildly decreased or normal	Lower than antigen	Normal	Variable	Normal distribution
2N	Normal	Normal	Decreased	Present using 1 mg ristocetin	Normal distribution
3	Severely decreased (< 10%)	Severely decreased (< 10%)	Severely decreased (< 10%)	Absent	Undetectable

*Result interpretation subject to ABO group (see table on page 38).

VWD primary profile limitations

- VWF is an acute phase reactant that rises during physical stress, pregnancy, hemorrhage, acute infection, estrogen therapy, and exercise. Normal laboratory results must be repeated if there is strong clinical suspicion for VWD based on personal or family history of bleeding.
- Some experts test women between the 5th and the 7th day of the menstrual cycle, the "VWF nadir."

VWF Level Varies by Blood Group (18)

Blood Group	Mean VWF	Range
O	75%	36–157%
A	105%	48–234%
B	117%	57–241%
AB	123%	64–238%

VWF Follow-Up Testing

- Ristocetin-induced platelet aggregation (RIPA), also called the ristocetin response curve, is used when VWD type 2B is suspected. In VWD type 2B, there is a disproportional decrease in VWF activity relative to VWF concentration. Platelets in type 2B VWD aggregate in response to 0.5 mg/mL ristocetin, a smaller concentration than the 1.0 mg/mL that activates normal platelets.
- VWF multimeric analysis is a specialized assay requiring SDS-polyacrylamide gel electrophoresis. Multimeric patterns distinguish among qualitative defects such as subtypes 2A and 2B. Multimeric analysis is unnecessary when type 1 or type 3 VWD is apparent from the primary profile.

VWD Treatment Options

Desmopressin (DDAVP)

- Useful in types 1, 2A, and 2M, because it releases intracellular stores of VWF from platelets and endothelial cells, increasing its plasma concentration
- Optimal dose of DDAVP is 0.3 µg/kg to a limit of 28 µg total dose in 15–30 mL of saline
- Given by slow IV push or drip over 15–30 minutes, or intranasally
- Peak VWF release effect of DDAVP is achieved in 30–60 minutes
- Half-life of released VWF is 12 hours

Fibrinolysis inhibitors

- EACA (Amicar) and Tranexamic acid
- Useful in dental and urinary tract procedures as topical therapy

Plasma-derived VWF concentrates

- Humate–P® is most commonly used and is approved for VWD only; Alphanate® is also an option
- Vials labeled with the number of units of factor VIII and VWF (also called ristocetin cofactor)

Calculating VWF concentrate dose

The normal level of VWF is roughly 50–150%, or 0.5–1.5 U/mL of plasma, depending on blood type (see table on previous page). A level of 50% is regarded as effectively hemostatic under normal conditions, although for major surgery one may aim for a higher level. The formula for computing the first, or loading, dose is:

$$\text{Dose in U} = (\text{desired activity} - \text{current activity}) \times PV$$

where:

- U is units, defined as amount per mL of plasma (1 U/mL = 100% activity)

- Desired activity is therapeutic level to be achieved
- Current VWF level is measured using the VWF antigen assay or VWF activity if a type 2
- PV is plasma volume in mL computed as follows:
    - PV = Blood volume × (1 − HCT)
    - Blood volume is calculated based on body type (see table below) and patient weight in kilograms (1 lb. = 0.453 kg)

Blood Volume by Body Type

Blood Volume Multiplier	Body Type
70 mL/kg	Slim
60 mL/kg	Obese
50 mL/kg	Morbidly obese

The maintenance dosage is 50% of the loading or initial dosage and is administered 12 hours after the first dosage. Subsequent dosages are administered at 12-hour intervals and are monitored by repeat VWF assays collected just prior to the next dose, called the trough level.

Example for calculating factor concentrate dosage

A woman with type 3 VWD arrives with an acute abdominal bleed. Her initial laboratory results:

- VWF activity   <1%
- VWF antigen   <1%
- Factor VIII activity   <1%
- Hematocrit   30%

She weighs 132 lbs and is 4'11" tall, moderately obese; blood volume multiplier is 60 mg/kg.

1. Compute blood volume:
   132 lb × 0.453 lb/kg = 60 kg
   BV = 60 kg × 60 mL/kg = 3600 mL

2. Compute plasma volume:
   PV = 3600 mL × (1 − .30) = 2520 mL
3. Compute dosage to achieve a peak of 50% VWF activity (0.5 U/mL):
   Dose in U = (0.5 U − 0 U) × 2520
   Dose = 1260 U
4. She is given an initial dose of approximately 1260 U of VWF in the form of Humate-P® and subsequent maintenance doses of approximately 630 U. VWF concentration should remain between 25 and 50% and dosage adjustments should follow factor levels.

Scurvy

Diagnosing scurvy and treating with vitamin C (19)

The diagnosis of scurvy requires a high index of suspicion. In western countries, the incidence appears to be on the rise. Populations at risk include the elderly, chronic alcoholics, diet faddists, the mentally ill, and patients who have cancer or malabsorption or who are on renal dialysis. The symptoms of scurvy are weakness, lassitude, depression, arthralgias, petechiae, perifollicular hemorrhage ("corkscrew hairs"), follicular hyperkeratosis, purpura, ecchymoses, gingival swelling, hemorrhage, halitosis, poor wound healing, and loss of teeth. Typical plaque-like ecchymoses of the lower extremities may also be present.

Adults should receive a loading dose of 100 mg of vitamin C 3–5 times a day up to 4 grams, followed by 100 mg/day. Infants and children should receive 10–25 mg 3 times a day. Symptoms should disappear within 3–5 days.

Congenital Single Factor Deficiencies (Hemophilias)

Hemophilia A and B are classified as mild (factor level of 5–20%), moderate (1–5%) or severe (<1%), based on the factor activity. They are clinically indistinguishable and inherited in an X-linked pattern. Hemophilia A is 4 times more common than hemophilia B, and 80% of patients have the severe form. There is a direct correlation between the plasma levels of factors VIII and IX and bleeding. Thus, factor replacement is often necessary to prevent (as in surgery) or treat hemorrhage.

Calculating factor VIII concentrate dosage

The normal level of factor VIII is 50–186% or 0.5–1.86 U/mL. Effective therapeutic levels vary from 30–100% depending on the clinical condition of the patient. The formula for computing the first or loading dose of factor is the same as that for VWF:

$$\text{Dose in U} = (\text{desired activity} - \text{current activity}) \times PV$$

where:

- U is units, defined as amount per mL of plasma (1 U/mL = 100%)
- Desired activity is therapeutic level to be achieved
- Current activity is measured using the factor VIII activity assay
- PV is plasma volume in mL computed as follows:

$$PV = \text{blood volume} \times (1 - HCT)$$

It is advisable to check the peak factor VIII level after the loading dose by collecting a sample approximately 15 minutes after the infusion of the factor. If the desired activity was achieved, 50% of the initial dose should be administered 8–12 hours later. Immediately prior to the second dose, another factor level assay helps to estimate the in vivo half-life of factor VIII and guides the calculation of subsequent doses. A bleeding patient is likely to require larger doses than someone who is clinically stable. Changes in hematocrit will also affect the appropriate dose at any given time.

Factor VIII Concentrates

Plasma-derived products

- Indicated for patients who have previously received plasma products or who have hepatitis B (HBV), hepatitis C (HCV), or human immunodeficiency virus (HIV) infection or positive serology
- Safe: after millions of units used, no evidence of viral transmission per Centers for Disease Control long-term surveillance (20)
- Equivalent choices include Monarc-M®, Hemofil-M®, Monoclate-P®, or Koate-HP®; all are labeled with factor VIII U per vial

Products prepared using recombinant technology

- Indicated for previously untreated patients (PUPs), those who have never been exposed to plasma products, or those whose previous treatment or serology status is unknown
- Equivalent choices include Kogenate®, Helixate®, Recombinate®, or Bioclate®; all are labeled with factor VIII U per vial

Calculating factor IX concentrate dosage

- Compute factor IX dosage as for VWF or factor VIII but double the initial dosage, because 50% of factor IX distributes to extravascular space.
- The maintenance dosage is 50% of the loading or initial dosage and is administered 24 hours after the first dose, reflecting the half-life of factor IX. Monitor factor activity as described for factor VIII above.

Factor IX Concentrates

Plasma-derived products

- Safe; indicated for patients who have previously received plasma products or who have HBV, HCV, or HIV infection or positive serology
- Equivalent choices include Alpha Nine SD® or Mononine®; labeled with factor IX U per vial

Products prepared using recombinant technology

- Indicated for previously untreated patients (PUPs), those who have never been exposed to plasma products, or those whose previous treatment is unknown
- BeneFIX®

Determining the Plasma Factor VIII or IX Activity from the PTT

When the factor assay is unavailable, such as during nights and weekends, plasma factor VIII or IX activity may be estimated using the PTT. In each laboratory, technologists may prepare correlations between PTT and factors VIII or IX (sensitivity curves). Because these correlations are specific for each reagent, they vary among laboratories and with reagent lot changes. PTT estimation of the degree of factor deficiency is valid only when the PT is normal, ruling out the presence of concomitant vitamin K deficiency or liver disease (not rare in patients infected with HCV). The PTT is seldom prolonged beyond 80 seconds in a single factor deficiency when the PT is normal. If the PTT is normal, the patient does not need factor replacement and another reason for the bleeding is likely.

Therapy Options for Factor Inhibitors

Up to 30% of severe hemophilia A patients develop factor VIII inhibitors (alloantibodies) after a few doses of factor VIII, rendering concentrate therapy ineffective. Adults who have never had a detectable inhibitor are unlikely to develop one. An inhibitor is suspected when the response to factor VIII concentrates is much less than predicted by the dose calculation (peak and/or trough levels).

Only 2–3% of hemophilia B patients develop anti-IX inhibitors. In rare instances, non-hemophilics may develop autoimmune factor VIII inhibitors, causing acquired hemophilia. To establish the presence of a factor inhibitor, order a PTT mixing study (see "Guidelines for the Management of Bleeding"). If there is no correction in the mixing study, a quantitative Bethesda assay will determine the relative concentration of inhibitor. In the presence of an inhibitor, treatment options include the following:

Activated Prothrombin Complex Concentrates (APCCs): FEIBA FH®, Autoplex T®

FEIBA dosages in U/kg (per manufacturer recommendations)

- Joint bleeding: 50 U/kg every 12 hours
- Mucous membrane bleeding: 50 U/kg every 6 hours
- Muscle bleeding: 100 U/kg every 12 hours

FEIBA may induce DIC, therefore:

- May not exceed 200 U/kg/24 hours
- Infusion or injection rate must not exceed 2 U/kg/minute

There is no test to monitor FEIBA. The patient's clinical response is the only guide; for example, monitor the size of the hematoma.

Activated Recombinant Factor VII (NovoSeven®)

- Effective alternative for inhibitor patients who do not respond to FEIBA
- Cost is ~$1/μg

- May be useful in patients with major bleeding associated with war-farin overdose or liver failure who require fast hemostasis
- For patients with factor VIII inhibitor: 90–120 µg/kg every 2–3 hours
- For other indications: 25–35 µg/kg once or every 6 hours (empiric dose—not determined in clinical trials).

Other Congenital Single-Factor Deficiencies

Patients with deficiencies of prothrombin or factors VII or X are rare, but may also present with spontaneous bleeding or bleeding during invasive procedures. The assayed plasma activity for factor VII does not correlate with risk or severity of bleeding, but the activities of prothrom-bin and factor X do. Besides FFP as a source of these factors, two types of prothrombin complex concentrates are available for these patients—and they are the products of choice.

Prothrombin Complex Concentrates (PCCs)

Amount of each factor per vial is relative to the number of units of fac-tor IX. *For example, there are 148 units of prothrombin per 100 units of factor IX in Profilnine HT.* The vials may be labeled with factor IX units only.

Prothrombin Complex Concentrates

Name	Factor II	Factor VII	Factor IX	Factor X
Profilnine HT®	148	11	100	64
Bebulin®	120	13	100	139

Steps in Using Factor Concentrates (Summary)

- Confirm coagulopathy diagnosis
- Determine current indication for factor replacement
- Select product:
    - Plasma-derived factors VIII or IX
    - Recombinant factors VIII or IX

- Bypass products for patients with factor VIII inhibitors
- Von Willebrand factor

- Assess availability of product in inventory
- Calculate dosage based on clinical indication
- Establish treatment frequency (dosing interval)
- Estimate expected number of repeat treatments required
- Determine laboratory monitoring by plasma factor level

  - Precise time interval
  - Frequency of testing

Guidelines for Management of Platelet Disorders

Platelet Count Ranges and Thrombocytopenia (21)

$150–400 \times 10^9/L$ Reference interval; $<150 \times 10^9/L$ is thrombocytopenia

$50–150 \times 10^9/L$ Bleeding unexpected, may imply qualitative platelet disorder

$10–50 \times 10^9/L$ Bleeding may follow trauma, surgery, or dental extraction

$<10 \times 10^9/L$ Spontaneous bleeding may require therapy

Thrombocytopenia: the most common cause of bleeding

- Inherited (multiple types) (22)
- Marrow hypoplasia: chemotherapy, drug sequelae, ethanol
- Immune-mediated platelet consumption: acute and chronic autoimmune thrombocytopenic purpura, drug-induced, neonatal alloimmune thrombocytopenia, post-transfusion purpura
- Non-immune mediated platelet consumption: TTP, HUS, DIC, HIT, type 2B VWD

Thrombocytosis: Platelet count $>400 \times 10^9/L$

- Reactive thrombocytosis with normal platelets: hemorrhage, surgery, iron deficiency anemia, inflammation; no bleeding risk; should be $<1 \times 10^{10}/L$
- Myeloproliferative disorders with abnormal platelets: essential thrombocythemia, chronic myelogenous leukemia, polycythemia vera; may cause thrombosis or bleeding

Platelet Diameter and Morphology

2.5–4 μm diameter	Average normal diameter
>7 μm diameter	Giant platelets imply myeloproliferative disorder, myelodysplastic syndrome, May-Hegglin anomaly
Gray platelets	Slightly enlarged gray platelets seen in Bernard-Soulier syndrome or α-granule deficiency (gray platelet syndrome)
Platelet clumps	Clotting due to improper specimen management or agglutination due to EDTA-dependent antibody
Platelet satellitism	Artifact of EDTA-dependent antibody

Qualitative Platelet Abnormalities (23)

These disorders may be diagnosed by abnormal platelet aggregation results, whereas platelet counts may be normal.

Congenital storage pool deficiency: dense granules

- Normal platelet dense granules store ADP, ATP, calcium, pyrophosphate, and serotonin, and release these during activation.
- Dense granule deficiency in non-albinos may be caused by an autosomal dominant inability to package the normal contents despite producing normal granules. Platelet counts are normal.
- Moderate thrombocytopenia with reduced dense granule distribution diagnosed by electron microscopy
  - *Hermansky-Pudlak* and *Chediak-Higashi* syndromes are rare autosomal recessive disorders with oculocutaneous albinism
  - *Wiskott-Aldrich* syndrome, an X-linked recessive disorder, is characterized by severe eczema

Congenital storage pool deficiency: α granules

- The α granules store coagulation factors, platelet-derived growth factor (PDGF), and platelet factor 4. They provide the granular appearance of platelets by light microscopy.

- Gray platelet syndrome is the absence of α granules; the platelets are large and pale on Wright-stained smears. Patients experience thrombocytopenia and moderate lifelong bleeding.

Acquired storage pool deficiency: myeloproliferative disorders or myelodysplastic syndromes

Platelets in these diseases show reduced α granules and dense granules, abnormal membranes, and they vary in size and count. Patients may present with mild to moderate bleeding, although thrombosis is also a risk. Platelet aggregometry may be used to predict clinical bleeding.

Platelet receptor defects

Following is a table of platelet membrane receptors and their defective state, which may be associated with mucocutaneous bleeding. These may be detected by platelet aggregometry.

Receptor	Function	Agonist	Defect
GP Ib/V/IX	VWF binding	Ristocetin	Bernard-Soulier syndrome
GP IIb/IIIa	Fibrinogen and VWF binding	ADP, collagen, epinephrine	Glanzmann's thrombasthenia

Metabolic pathway defects

Defects in cyclooxygenase and thromboxane synthetase result in decreased thromboxane A_2 production and poor platelet secretion despite normal granule distribution. These are called platelet release or secretion defects. They resemble the effect of aspirin on cyclooxygenase, hence the term "aspirin-like disorders." These are detected by a reduced aggregation response to arachidonic acid agonist.

Other acquired qualitative platelet conditions

Multiple myeloma, cardiopulmonary bypass surgery, liver disease, and uremia are all associated with reduced platelet function.

Drugs with Anti-Platelet Activity

Platelets are inhibited by many common drugs such as aspirin, non-steroidal anti-inflammatory drugs (NSAIDs), various antibiotics, herbs, garlic, and vitamin E (among many others). Specific platelet inhibitors include clopidogrel and ticlopidine, which block ADP receptors, and abciximab, eptifibatide, and tirofiban, which bind to the IIb/IIIa receptors. Complications of some of these drugs include immune and thrombotic thrombocytopenic purpura.

Platelet Aggregometry

Platelet aggregometry is a qualitative functional test performed on whole blood or platelet-rich plasma. An agonist (platelet activator) is added to the suspension and a dynamic measure of platelet clumping is recorded. ATP release is simultaneously assayed using a luminescent marker.

Expected Aggregation and Secretion Results for Aspirin, Release Defect, Membrane Defect, or Storage Pool Disorder using a Variety of Agonists

Agonist	Aspirin or Release Defect	Membrane Defect	Storage Pool Deficiency
Thrombin	Normal secretion and aggregation	Normal secretion and aggregation	Decreased secretion and aggregation
Arachidonic acid	Decreased secretion and aggregation	Normal secretion and aggregation	Decreased secretion and aggregation
ADP, epinephrine, and collagen	Decreased secretion and aggregation	Decreased secretion and aggregation	Decreased secretion and aggregation

Platelet Concentrate Therapy (21)

Two types of platelet components are used for platelet replacement:

1. "Platelets," also called random donor platelets, are pooled concentrates prepared from whole blood donations by centrifugation. A pool usually consists of 6 units, providing an adult dose of 1 unit/10 kg of body weight. Each random unit contains at least 5×10^{10} platelets.
2. "Platelets, apheresis," or single donor platelets, are prepared by apheresis of one donor and contain a minimum of 3×10^{11} platelets.

Therapeutic platelet transfusions treat bleeding due to defects in platelet production or platelet function. Transfusion of platelets is contraindicated for diseases involving thrombotic consumption of platelets, including TTP, HUS, and HIT. Platelet transfusions are not usually effective in immune-mediated thrombocytopenias, although there may be some benefit in life-threatening situations such as central nervous system bleeding.

Recommended Triggers for the Use of Platelet Transfusions

Stable oncohematological recipient, lumbar puncture in stable pediatric leukemia, thrombocytopenia secondary to GPIIb/IIIa receptor inhibitors	10×10^9/L
Bone marrow aspiration and biopsy	20×10^9/L
Gastrointestinal endoscopy in cancer	$20–40 \times 10^9$/L
DIC, fiber-optic bronchoscopy in a bone marrow transplant recipient	$20–50 \times 10^9$/L
Neonatal alloimmune thrombocytopenia	30×10^9/L
Major surgery in leukemia, thrombocytopenia due to massive transfusion, invasive procedure in cirrhosis	50×10^9/L
Cardiopulmonary bypass	$50–60 \times 10^9$/L
Liver biopsy, non-bleeding premature infant, neurosurgery	$50–100 \times 10^9$/L

Ideally, the effectiveness of platelet transfusions will be confirmed by bleeding cessation. If there are no complicating factors affecting response, such as hemorrhage, fever, or splenomegaly, a single unit of random platelets should increase the recipient's platelet count by $5-10 \times 10^9$/L, and a unit of apheresis platelets should increase the count by $30-50 \times 10^9$/L. Many multi-transfused patients do not show the expected increment after platelet transfusion. The most common method to determine if the recipient is refractory to platelets is to measure the platelet count within one hour post-transfusion and calculate the corrected count increment (CCI):

$$CCI = \frac{(\text{Post-transfusion PLT ct} - \text{Pre-transfusion PLT ct}) \times \text{body area (m}^2)}{\text{Number of platelets transfused (multiples of } 10^{11})}$$

A CCI above 7.5×10^9/L indicates an adequate response to platelet transfusion. A CCI below 7.5×10^9/L suggests immune-mediated clearance via antibodies to human leukocyte antigens (HLA) or platelet-specific antigens, and is the basis for the procurement of cross-matched platelets for subsequent transfusions.

Treating Uremic Platelet Dysfunction with Red Blood Cells

Uremic hemorrhage results from platelet abnormalities secondary to kidney failure. While platelet transfusions may be used, they are not very effective. CRYO may be helpful but packed *red blood cells* are the treatment of choice, particularly if the patient is anemic. A target hematocrit of 30% has been shown to improve platelet function in uremic patients.

Thrombotic Thrombocytopenic Purpura (TTP) and the VWF-Cleaving Protease Assay

Patients with TTP have circulating ultra-large molecular weight VWF multimers. In many of them, this appears to be the consequence of deficiency of the VWF-cleaving protease (ADAMTS-13), responsible for the normal digestion of endothelial cell-secreted VWF. Lack of enzyme activity is most commonly the consequence of an autoantibody in the acquired form of TTP. In rare cases, TTP is familial and due to congenital absence of ADAMTS-13. In adults, HUS is indistinguishable from TTP. In children, bacterial toxins cause classical HUS, and the VWF-cleaving protease activity is normal. Although measurement of ADAMTS-13 activity is helpful in the diagnosis of TTP, the current assay is complex and the turnaround time is several days. Furthermore, a normal result does not rule out TTP. Thus, TTP-HUS is a clinical diagnosis that demands emergent plasmapheresis. To test for ADAMTS-13 activity and its inhibitor, always collect a blood specimen prior to starting the first plasma exchange.

References

1. Clinical Laboratory and Standards Institute. Collection, transport, and processing of blood specimens for testing plasma-based coagulation assays; approved guideline, 4th Ed. Document H21-A4. Wayne, PA: CLSI, 2003.

2. Colman RW, Clowes AM, George JN, Goldhaber SZ, Marder VJ. Overview of hemostasis. In: Colman RW, Clowes AM, George JN, Goldhaber SZ, Marder VJ, eds. Hemostasis and thrombosis: basic principles and clinical practice, 5th Ed. Philadelphia, PA: Lippincott Williams & Wilkins, 2006.

3. Bounameaux, H. Overview of venous thromboembolism. In: Colman RW, Clowes AM, George JN, Goldhaber SZ, Marder VJ, eds. Hemostasis and thrombosis: basic principles and clinical practice, 5th Ed. Philadelphia, PA: Lippincott Williams & Wilkins, 2006.

4. Brandt JT, Triplett DA, Alving B, Scharrer I. Criteria for the diagnosis of lupus anticoagulants: an update. On behalf of the Subcommittee on Lupus Anticoagulant/Antiphospholipid Antibody of the Scientific and Standardisation Committee of the ISTH. Thromb Haemost 1995;74: 1185–90.

5. Proceedings of the 8th International Symposium on Antiphospholipid Antibodies. Sapporo, Japan, 6–9 October 1998. Lupus 1998;7: S1–234.

6. Levine JS, Branch W, Rauch J. The antiphospholipid syndrome. N Engl J Med 2002;346:752–63.

7. Heit JA. Epidemiology of venous thromboembolism. In: Colman RW, Clowes AM, George JN, Goldhaber SZ, Marder VJ, eds. Hemostasis and thrombosis: basic principles and clinical practice, 5th Ed. Philadelphia, PA: Lippincott Williams & Wilkins, 2006.

8. Bauer K. Hypercoagulable states. Hematology 2005;10(Suppl 1):39.

9. Itakura H. Racial disparities in risk factors for thrombosis. Curr Opin Hematol 2005;12:364–9.

10. Ansell J, Hirsch J, Poller L, Bussey H, Jacobson A, Hylek E. The pharmacology and management of the vitamin K antagonists: the Seventh ACCP Conference on Antithrombotic and Thrombolytic Therapy. Chest 2004;126:204S–33S.

11. Harrington RA, Becker RC, Ezekowitz M, Meade TW, O'Connor CM, Vorchheimer DA, et al. Antithrombotic therapy for coronary artery disease: the Seventh ACCP Conference on Antithrombotic and Thrombolytic Therapy. Chest 2004;126:513S–48S.

12. Hirsh J, Raschke R. Heparin and low-molecular-weight heparin: the Seventh ACCP Conference on Antithrombotic and Thrombolytic Therapy. Chest 2004;126:188S–203S.

13. Warkentin TE, Greinacher A. Heparin-induced thrombocytopenia: recognition, treatment, and prevention: the Seventh ACCP Conference on Antithrombotic and Thrombolytic Therapy. Chest 2004;126:311S–37S.

14. Liu MC, Kessler CM. A systematic approach to the bleeding patient. In: Kitchens CS, Alving BM, Kessler CM, eds. Consultative hemostasis and thrombosis. Philadelphia, PA: WB Saunders, 2002.

15. Franchini M, Gandini G, Di Paolantonio T, Mariani G. Acquired hemophilia A: a concise review. Am J Hematol 2005;80:55–63.

16. Kitchens C. Disseminated intravascular coagulation. In: Kitchens CS, Alving BM, Kessler CM, eds. Consultative hemostasis and thrombosis. Philadelphia, PA: WB Saunders, 2002.

17. Rick ME. Von Willebrand disease. In: Kitchens CS, Alving BM, Kessler CM, eds. Consultative hemostasis and thrombosis. Philadelphia, PA: WB Saunders, 2002.

18. Gill JC, Endres-Brooks J, Bauer PJ, Marks WJ Jr, Montgomery RR. The effect of ABO blood group on the diagnosis of von Willebrand disease. Blood 1987;69:1691–5.

19. De Luna RH, Colley BJ 3rd, Smith K, Divers SG, Rinehart J, Marques MB. Scurvy: an often forgotten cause of bleeding. Am J Hematol 2003;74:85–7.

20. Centers for Disease Control and Prevention (CDC). Blood safety monitoring among persons with bleeding disorders—United States, May 1998–June 2002. MMWR 2003;51:1152–4.

21. Angiolillo A, Abu-Ghosh AM, Davenport V, Cairo MS. General aspects of thrombocytopenia, platelet transfusions, and thrombopoeitic growth factors. In: Kitchens CS, Alving BM, Kessler CM, eds.

Consultative hemostasis and thrombosis. Philadelphia, PA: WB Saunders, 2002.

22. Balduini CL, Iolascon A, Savoia A. Inherited thrombocytopenias: from genes to therapy. Haematologica 2002;87:860–80.

23. Rao K. Disorders of platelet function. In: Kitchens CS, Alving BM, Kessler CM, eds. Consultative hemostasis and thrombosis. Philadelphia, PA: WB Saunders, 2002.

INDEX

A

acquired thrombophilia, 14
activated prothrombin complex concentrate (APCC), 45
aggregometry, 1–2, 8, 51, 52
anticardiolipin (ACL) testing, 6, 15, 16, 18, 19
anticoagulant therapy monitoring, 9
  guidelines, 21–28
antiphospholipid syndrome (APS), 19
Arixtra®, see fondaparinux

B

Bethesda assay, 8, 31, 45
bleeding, 31, 36, 49
  acquired vs. congenital, 29–30, 31
bleeding disorder assays, 7–9
blood components, 32–34
blood specimen, 1
  collection, 1

instructions to maintain integrity of, 1–2
quality of, 1

C

coagulation factor inhibitors, 8
coagulation mechanism, 11
  controls, 12
coagulopathy, 29, 30, 34, 46
  tests to establish presence of, 30
corrected count increment (CCI), 54
Coumadin®, see warfarin
cryoprecipitate (CRYO), 33–34, 54

D

desmopressin (DDAVP), 39
dilute Russell viper venom time (DRVVT), 10, 16, 18
direct thrombin inhibitors (DTIs), 9, 27, 28